I0429146

Paleo Diet for Beginners

Paleo Diet for Beginners Who Want to Get a Healthier Life

Sarah Sparrow

PUBLISHED BY:
Sarah Sparrow
Copyright © 2014

Disclaimer

The information contained in this book is for general information purposes only. The information is provided by the authors and while we endeavor to keep the information up to date and correct, we make no representations or warranties of any kind, express or implied, about the completeness, accuracy, reliability, suitability or availability with respect to the book or the information, products, services, or related graphics contained in the book for any purpose. Any reliance you place on such information is therefore strictly at your own risk.

TABLE OF CONTENTS

Introduction

The Paleo Recipe Book for Beginners is your guide to a whole new way of eating and a cleaner, healthier life.

The recipes in the book have been carefully selected to ensure they are easy to make and adhere to Paleo guidelines. Simple items like Roast Chicken and Mashed Sweet Potatoes and Creamy Cauliflower Soup will give you that same home-cooked comfort that their non-Paleo counterparts as you transition into the Paleo World.

One of the challenges when starting out on the Paleo diet is figuring out how to snack on a Paleo Diet - it seems tricky but this book has the solution. The Paleo Recipe Book for Beginners starts off with 31 days of simple snack ideas like homemade Cashew Butter on Celery Boats, Zesty Salsa with Bacon Chips and Pumpkin Spice Smoothies

The second half of the book gives you 31 days of fantastic meal ideas. Paleo Spaghetti Noodles and Paleo Cauliflower Rice will become staples in your diet while delicious creations like Thai Coconut Curry and Tropical Chicken Skewers can take you on a weeknight taste adventure. The recipes have been carefully balanced to work with your body and you will see a difference in the way you look and feel within two weeks.

Expect more energy, glowing skin and a little kick in your step as you walk with your new found Paleo confidence.

Happy Paleo!

The Paleo Lifestyle

Paleo eating means making food choices that help our bodies make us look good and feel great.

The human body is an incredible machine that can work in optimal mode when we do not clog it up with foods that it was not designed to process such as legumes, dairy and grains. Once the body is working in optimal mode, we have more energy and it becomes healthier.

If we think about the foods our Paleolithic ancestors would have eaten we can determine what kinds of foods are natural for the body to process. Food that requires heavy processing would not have been eaten by our Paleo ancestors since present-day machinery and tools were not available then. People ate foods their bodies could process.

Today we have taken foods that cannot be broken down by the human body. Many health problems can be attributed by eating processed foods such as obesity, diabetes, heart problems, etc. The elimination of processed foods leads to weight loss within two weeks because the body is only ingesting foods that it needs and none of the gunk found in processed foods.

The Paleo lifestyle is about clean, healthy living and includes an array of natural good foods like vegetables, nuts, fruits and meats. These foods are packed full of nutrients the body needs to function and what's even better is the food choices leave you feeling full.

Paleo Food List

One of the big reasons the Paleo diet has so many followers is because the list of foods you are allowed to eat is long and the choices delicious. The following is a short list of foods you can eat and those you should avoid.

Vegetables

Vegetables are great sources of nutrients and should play a large part in your Paleo Diet, in addition to being healthy, they are also great substitutes for carbohydrates. The following is a short list of veggies you will likely be eating a lot more of:

Kale
Spinach
Broccoli
Tomatoes
Cauliflower
Carrots
Eggplant
Squash

Sweet Potatoes

Fruits
Fruits are full of good-for-you vitamins and are also Paleo-friendly, just remember not to go overboard on fruits that are very high on sugar like pineapple.

Blueberry
Cranberry
Strawberry
Pomegranate
Apple
Orange
Banana

Proteins
Protein is essential for our bodies and following in the footsteps of our Paleolithic ancestors, the best sources are meats, seafood and nuts. Try to purchase lean cuts of meat and remember to portion-control your nut consumption since they are high in fat.

Turkey
Beef
Chicken
Pork
Deer
Rabbit

Fish
Shrimp
Crab
Lobster
Mussels

Walnuts
Almonds
Cashews
Macadamia Nut
Pistachio

Foods to Eliminate

As a Paleo-eater you will need to eliminate all foods that our bodies were not designed to process including the following:

Legumes
Peanuts
Beans
Lentils

Grains
Bread
Wraps
Pasta
Rice

Dairy
Milk
Cheese
Yogurt
Ice cream

Sugar
Alcohol
Processed Foods

SNACKS

Roasted Red Pepper Hummus
Serves: 4
Prep Time: 10 minutes

Ingredients:
3 red bell peppers, seeded, quartered
1 cup Brazil nuts (soaked overnight)
4 cloves garlic, peeled
2 lemons, juiced
1 tsp salt
1 tsp paprika
Extra virgin olive oil

Directions:

1. Preheat oven to 400 degrees, coat baking tray with olive oil.
2. Place garlic on baking tray, cover with bell peppers, drizzle with olive oil and roast for 10 minutes.
3. Place all ingredients in food processor and mix until fairly smooth.
4. Enjoy with veggies of choice.

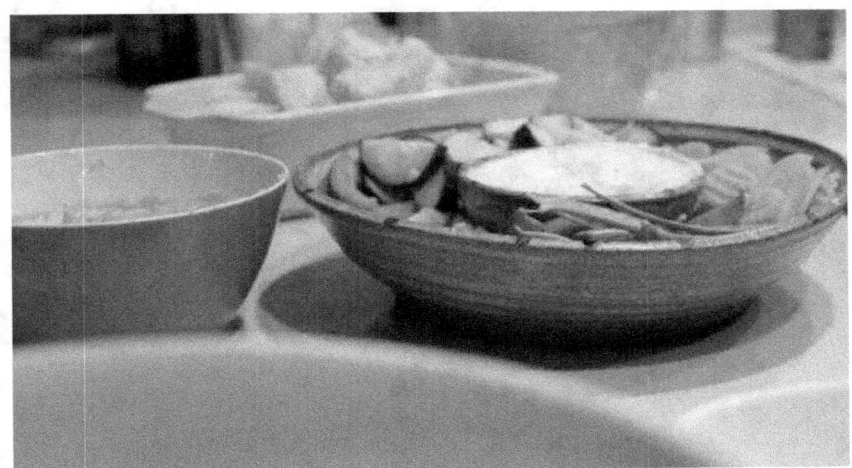

https://flic.kr/p/7g5e4C by timlewisnmCC BY-SA 2.0

Paleo Dill Dip

Serves: 4
Prep Time: 10 minutes

Ingredients:

1 egg
1/2 cup fresh dill, chopped
3/4 cup extra virgin olive oil
3 tsp lemon juice
1/4 tsp dry mustard
1/2 tsp salt
3 cups broccoli florets

Directions:

1. Crack egg into large mixing bowl.
2. Using a hand immersion blender, mix in the olive oil to the egg until mixture becomes thick.
3. Add remaining ingredients and mix for another minute.
4. Enjoy dip with broccoli florets or with celery and other vegetables

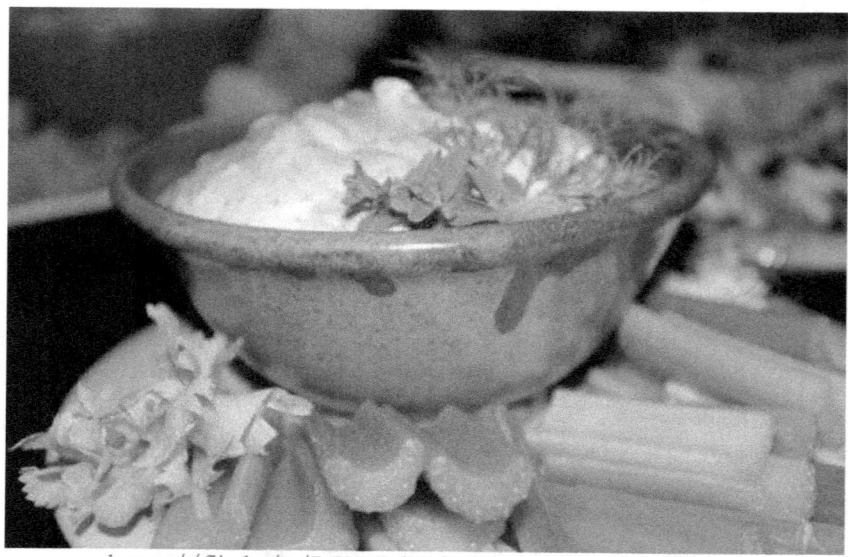

Sesame Crackers

Serves 2
Prep Time: 10 minutes

Ingredients:

1 cup almond flour
1 egg
¼ tsp salt
¼ cup sesame seeds

Directions:

1. Preheat oven to 325 degrees.
2. Toast sesame seeds in non-stick pan for 3-4 minutes.
3. Combine almond flour, egg, salt, knead dough.
4. Place baking paper on flat surface and roll out dough.

5. Place baking paper with dough on cookie sheet, sprinkle with sesame seeds and bake for 12 minutes.
6. Enjoy with lovely Paleo dips.

Dill Tuna Salad on Cucumber Coins

Serves: 1
Prep Time: 5 minutes

Ingredients:
500 g can Tuna (drain the liquid)
2 tbsp dill dip
¼ cup celery, finely chopped
½ tsp salt, pepper
½ English cucumber

Directions:
1. Combine all ingredients save cucumber.
2. Slice cucumber into ½ inch coins.
3. Scoop a little tuna on each coin and enjoy.

Cauliflower Hummus with Red Bell Dippers

Serves: 4
Prep Time: 10 minutes

Ingredients:
5 cups cauliflower florets
3 cloves garlic, peeled
1/2 cup walnuts, soaked overnight
1 tsp tahini (or 1 tsp almond butter)
1 lemon, juiced
1/2 tsp sea salt
1 tsp white pepper

2 large red bell peppers, seeded

Directions:
1. Place cauliflower in food processor and pulse until crumbly.
2. Add remaining ingredients until hummus is fairly smooth.
3. Slice red bell peppers into strips and serve with hummus.

Zesty Salsa and Bacon Chips

Serves: 2
Prep Time: 15 minutes

Ingredients:

Salsa
2 green bell peppers, seeded and quartered
1 onion, peeled, rough-chopped
2 tomatoes, diced
1 cup tomato purée
1/4 cup vinegar
1 tsp cumin
1 tsp oregano
1 tsp salt, black pepper
Bacon Chips
8 strips turkey bacon

Directions:

Salsa
Place veggies in food processor and chop.
Add remaining ingredients and mix until well-combined.
Refrigerate overnight.

Bacon Chips
Preheat oven to 375 degrees and place baking sheet on baking tray.
Place turkey slices on baking sheet and cook for 10 minutes or until crispy.

Garlic Zucchini Chips

Serves: 4
Prep Time: 10 minutes

Ingredients:

4 zucchinis
1/4 cup olive oil
4 cloves garlic
1 tsp salt

Directions:

1. Preheat oven to 375 degrees and lightly coat tray with olive oil.
2. Peel garlic and place in food processor and chop, until garlic turns into a chunky paste.
3. Add oil and salt to garlic and mix well.
4. Slice zucchini into translucent discs and place on baking tray.
5. Drizzle with garlic mixture and bake in oven for 10 minutes
6. Allow to cool before serving.

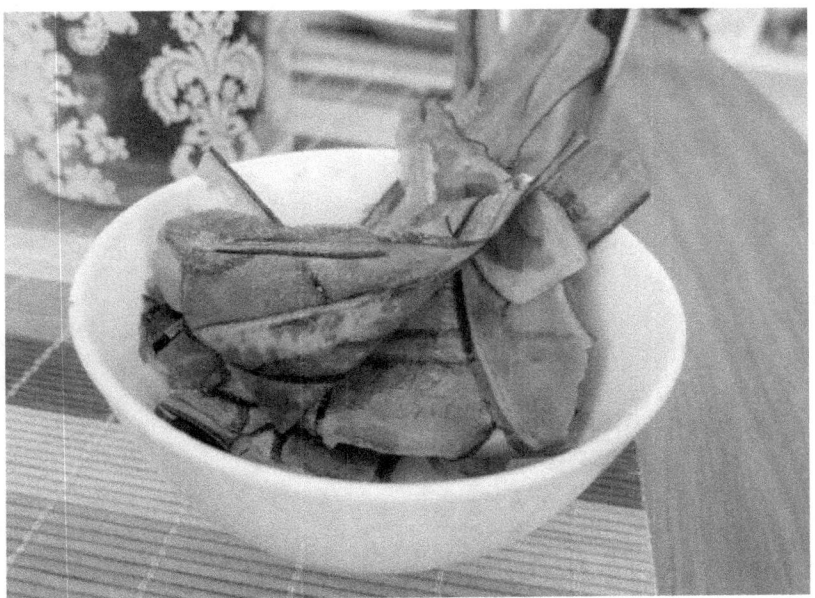

Eggplant Basil Snackers
Serves: 4
Prep Time: 10 minutes

Ingredients:
1 large eggplant
1/2 cup fresh basil, washed and chopped
1/4 cup extra virgin olive oil
4 cloves garlic, peeled and minced
1/4 cup walnuts
1 tsp salt

Directions:
1. Preheat oven to 375 degrees and lightly coat baking tray with olive oil.
2. Place walnut, basil, olive oil, garlic and salt in blender.
3. Mix until mixture turns to paste.
4. Slice eggplant into 1/2" slices and place on baking pan.
5. Brush eggplant slices with basil mixture.
6. Place in oven for 20 minutes.

Brussels Sprout Snackers

Serves: 4
Prep Time: 10 minutes

Ingredients:
1 lb Brussels sprouts
1 tsp each salt and pepper
1 tbsp garlic powder
1 tbsp rosemary
1 lemon, juiced
Extra virgin olive oil

Directions:
1. Preheat oven to 350 degrees and lightly coat roasting tray with olive oil.
2. Mix salt, pepper, garlic powder, rosemary and 4 tbsp olive oil in large bowl.
3. Chop Brussels sprouts in half and toss with olive oil mixture.
4. Place Brussels sprouts on baking tray and bake for 20 minutes, turning halfway.

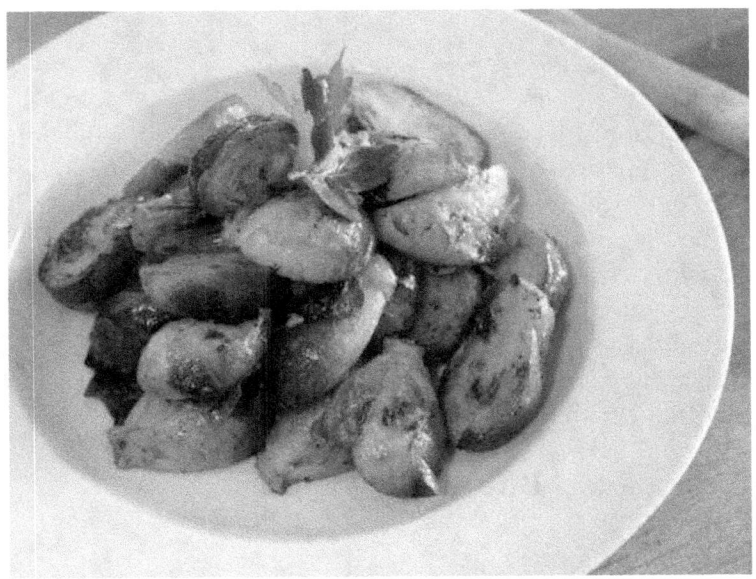

Toasted Almonds

Serves: 2
Prep Time: 5 minutes

Ingredients:
½ cup almonds
¼ tsp salt

Directions:
1. Place non-stick pan over medium heat.
2. Place almonds in pan and toast until fragrant.
3. Sprinkle with a little salt.

Egg on Grilled Avocado Slice

Serves: 1
Prep Time: 10 minutes

Ingredients:
1 avocado
1 egg
Extra virgin olive oil

Salt and pepper

Directions:
1. Bring pot of water to a boil, add egg and cook for five minutes, peel, set aside.
2. Pit and peel avocado, cut avocado into four flat slices and use one slice per serving, refrigerate unused slices.
3. Lightly coat grill pan with olive oil and heat.
4. Place one slice of avocado on pan and grill each side for a minute.
5. Slice egg vertically into three slices and place on avocado.
6. Sprinkle with salt, pepper as desired

Margherita Pizza Bites
Serves: 2
Prep Time: 10 minutes

Ingredients:
2 zucchinis
½ cup tomato puree
¼ cup chopped basil
¼ cup cashew, soaked overnight
1 tsp garlic salt
1 tsp black pepper
Extra virgin olive oil

Directions:
1. Preheat oven to 425 degrees and coat baking tray with olive oil.
2. Mix tomato, basil, salt, pepper, set aside.
3. Crush cashews in food processor until grainy.
4. Slice zucchini into ½" discs, place in baking tray.
5. Top zucchini slice with tomato mixture and a little cashew.
6. Bake in oven for 10 minutes

Bacon-Melon Bites
Serves: 2
Prep Time: 10 minutes

Ingredients:

1-1/2 cup melon, cubed
4 slices bacon

Directions:
1. Cook bacon in non-stick pan over medium heat, 3 minutes per side.
2. Slice bacon into quarters.
3. Using toothpicks, skewer one piece melon and bacon.

Cracked Pepper Wings

Serves: 6
Prep Time: 10 minutes

Ingredients:
1 lb chicken wings, skinless
1 lemon juiced
1 tsp cracked black pepper
1 tsp salt
2 tbsp extra virgin olive oil

Directions:
1. Set wings aside, mix remaining ingredients.
2. Marinate wings in mixture for 3 hours.
3. Preheat oven to 375 degrees
4. Place wings in baking dish and bake for 20 minutes, turning at halfway point

Rosemary Sweet Potato Fries

Serves: 1
Prep Time: 10 minutes

Ingredients:
1 sweet potato
½ tsp rosemary
½ tsp salt and coarse black pepper
Extra virgin olive oil

Directions:
1. Preheat oven to 400 degrees and coat baking tray with olive oil.

2. Slice sweet potato into fries and toss with 3 tbsp olive oil, rosemary, salt and pepper
3. Place on baking tray without overlapping, bake in oven for 20 minutes; turn half way   through cooking time.

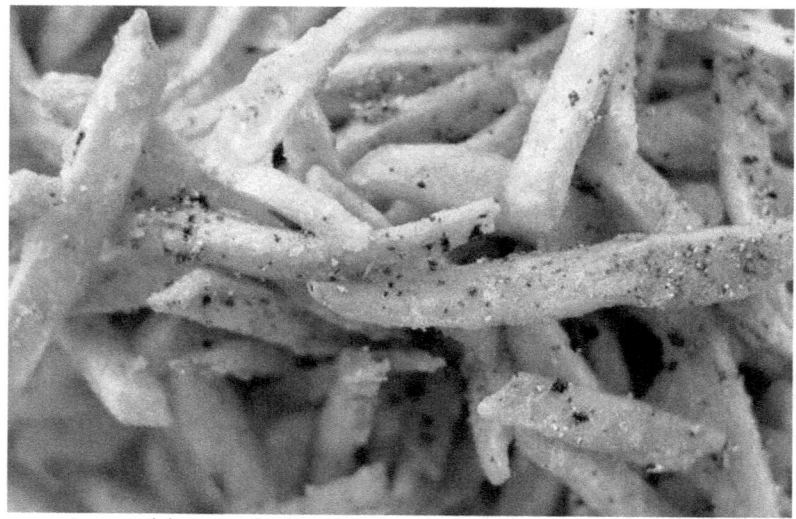

https://flic.kr/p/9z6Jer by Dean SebournCC BY 2.0

Bacon Green Beans

Serves: 2
Prep Time: 5 minutes

Ingredients:
2 cups green beans, stemmed
¼ cup bacon, crumbled
1 lemon, juiced
1 tablespoon of chopped almonds (optional)
Salt to taste

Directions:
1. Place green beans in steamer for 10 minutes.
2. Place bacon in skillet and cook until crispy, crumble.
3. Remove green beans from steamer (they should still be slightly firm), mix with lemon juice, bacon, almonds and salt.

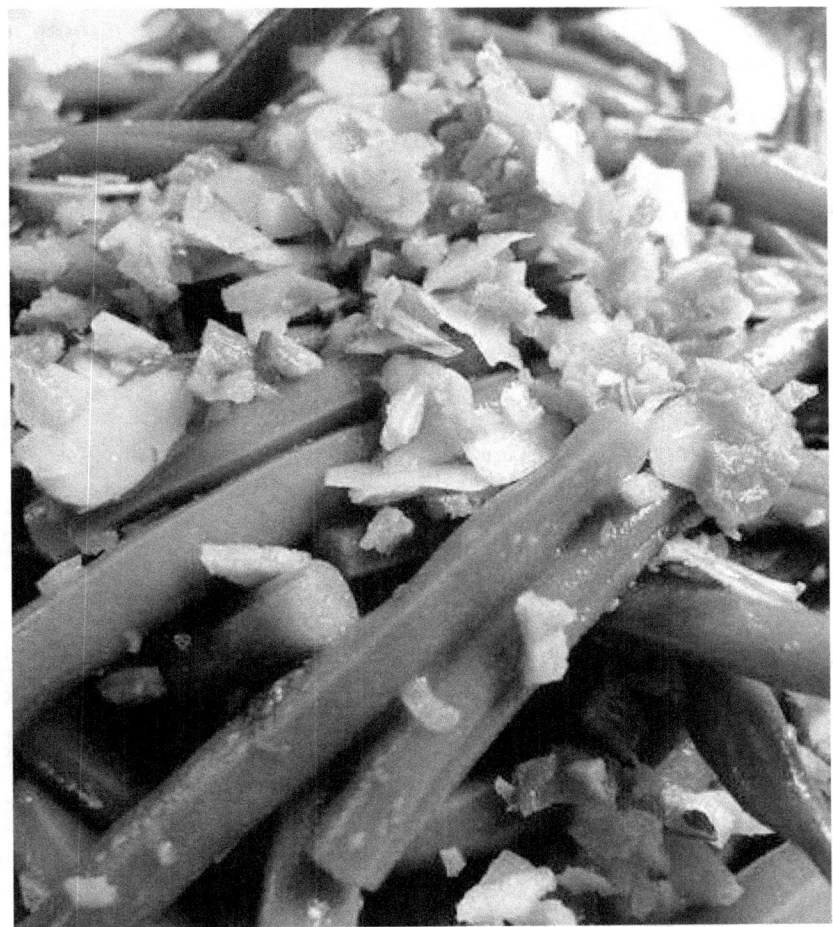

Cucumber Turkey Wraps

Serves: 2
Prep Time: 15 minutes

Ingredients:
1 cucumber, peeled
300 g organic deli Turkey slices

Directions:
1. Slice cucumber into long paper-thin strips.

2. Place turkey slice on cucumber slice and roll up, use toothpick to hold in place.

Homemade Almond Butter

Serves: 4
Prep Time: 10 minutes

Ingredients:
1 cup almonds, soaked overnight
1/2 tsp sea salt

Directions:
1. Peel almonds and place in food processor.
2. Add salt and blend until butter reaches desired consistency.
3. Enjoy with celery and carrot sticks or on apple slices

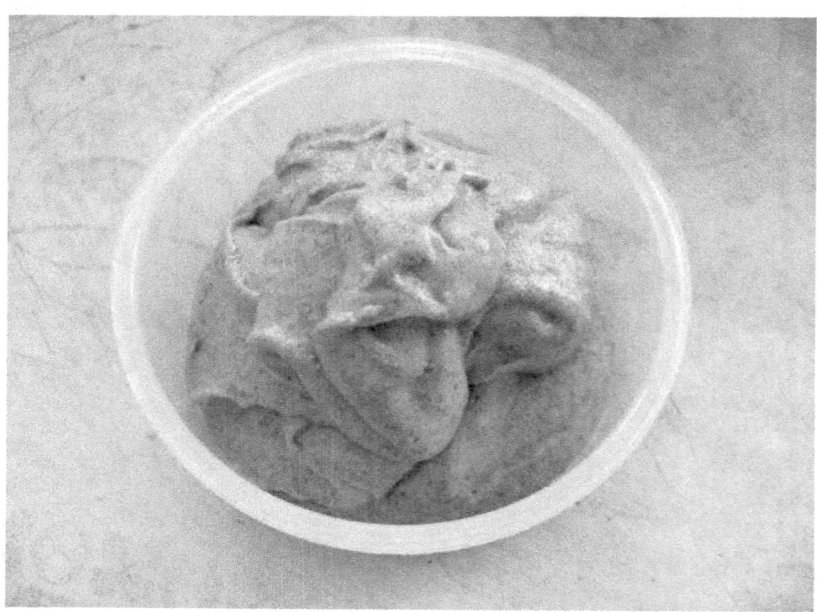

Banana Almond Butter Sandwich

Serves: 1
Prep Time: 5 minutes

Ingredients:
1 tbsp almond butter
1 banana

Directions:
1. Slice banana in half vertically, spread almond butter on each half.
2. Sandwich banana back together and slice in half horizontally.

Coconut Date Balls

Serves: 4
Prep Time: 10 minutes

Ingredients:
8 Medjool Dates, pitted
2 tbsp almond butter
¼ cup coconut, shredded

Directions:
1. Place dates and almond butter in food processor and mix.
2. Roll date mixture into small balls and roll in shredded coconut.
3. Refrigerate for two hours.

Decadent Cashew Nut Butter

Serves: 6
Prep Time: 10 minutes

Ingredients:
1/2 cup cashews, soaked overnight
1 tbsp molasses
1/2 tsp salt

Directions:
1. Mix ingredients in blender until smooth.
2. Enjoy with apple slices.

No-bake Nut Bars

Serves: 4
Prep Time: 10 minutes

Ingredients:

4 tbsp cashew butter
½ cup dried cranberries
½ cup almonds, crushed
½ cup flaxseed
2 tbsp coconut oil

Directions:

1. Line small baking tray with wax paper.
2. Mix ingredients and pat down in tray.
3. Refrigerate for four hours.

Celery Cashew Boats

Serves: 1
Prep Time: 5 minutes

Ingredients:

2 celery stalks
2 tbsp cashew butter
¼ cup raisins

Directions:

1. Fill celery stalks with cashew butter and sprinkle with raisins.

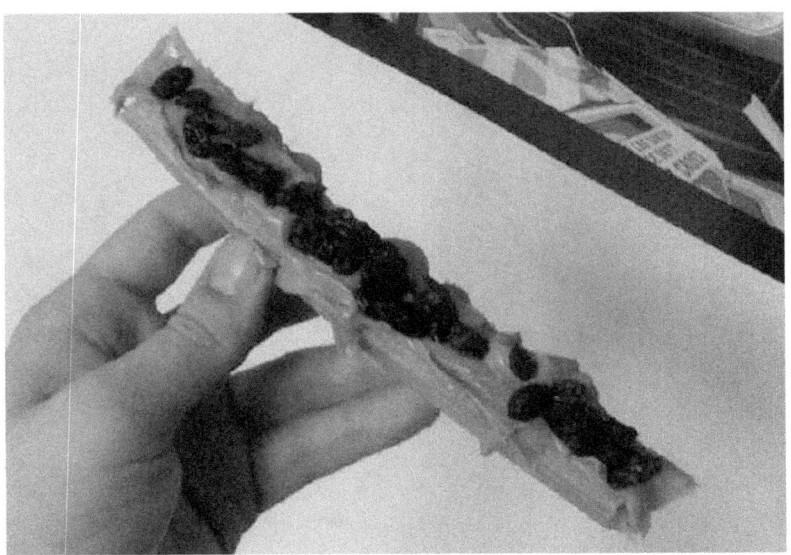

Banana Chips

Serves: 2
Prep Time: 10 minutes

Ingredients:
2 bananas
1 lemon, juiced

Directions:
1. Preheat oven to 200 degrees and line baking tray with parchment.
2. Slice banana into ¼" discs, sprinkle with lemon and place in baking tray.
3. Bake for one hour, set aside to cool and crisp.

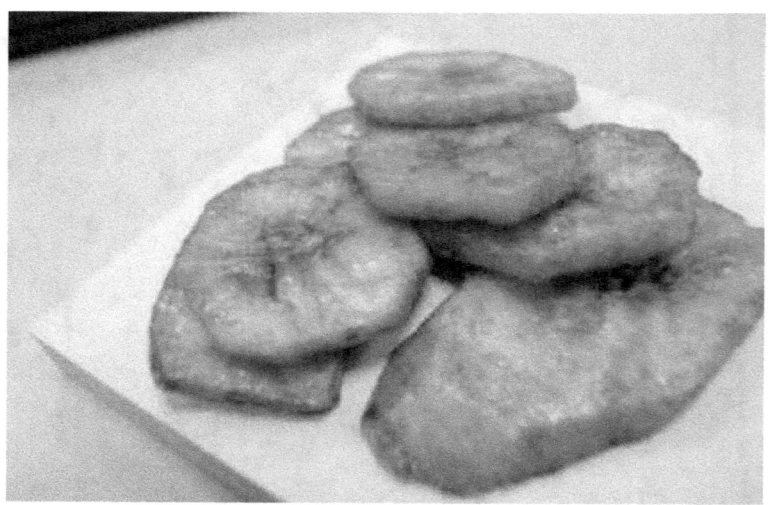

Strawberries with Pistachio Rain

Serves: 1
Prep Time: 5 minutes

Ingredients:
½ cup strawberries
¼ cup pistachio nuts, crushed

Directions:
1. Sprinkle pistachio over strawberries for light healthy snack or dessert.

Chocolate Bananasicles

Serves: 4
Prep Time: 15 minutes

Ingredients:
4 bananas
Dark chocolate (70% cocoa)

Directions:
1. Bring pot of water to boil.

2. Break up chocolate pieces and place in glass bowl that will fit over boiling water pot.
3. Place glass bowl over water bath, stir until chocolate is melted.
4. Dip peeled bananas in chocolate and place in freezer for 6 hours.

Raspberry Almond Smoothie

Serves: 1
Prep Time: 10 minutes

Ingredients:
1/2 cup almond milk
1/2 cup raspberries
1 cup ice

Directions:
Place ingredients in blender and mix until smooth.

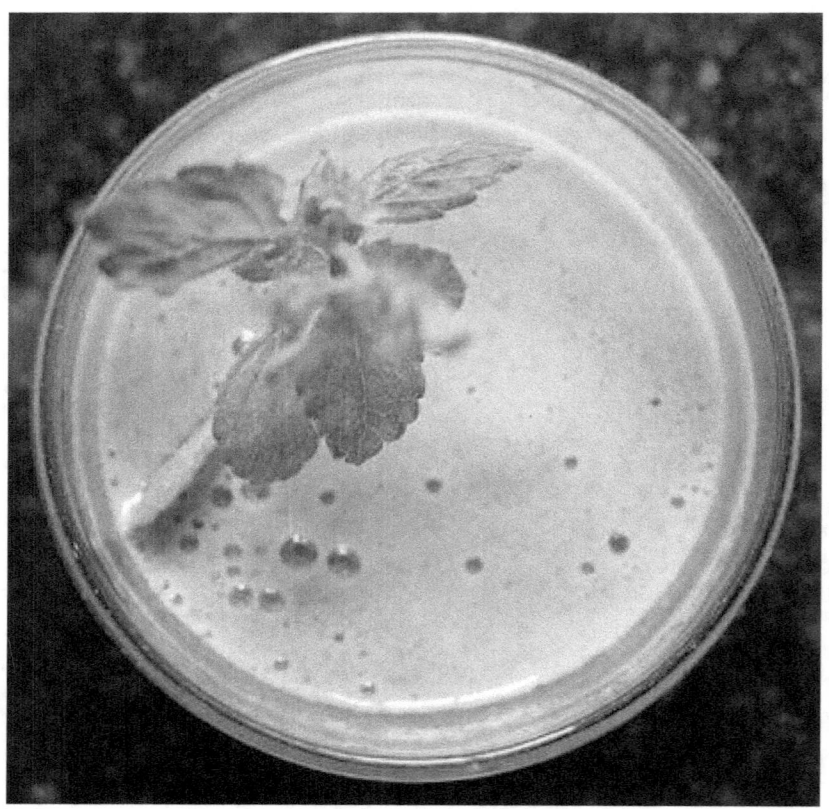

Strawberry Banana Smoothie
Serves: 2
Prep Time: 10 minutes

Ingredients:
½ cup strawberries
1 banana
½ cup almond milk
½ cup ice

Directions:
1. Place smoothie in blender and mix until smooth.

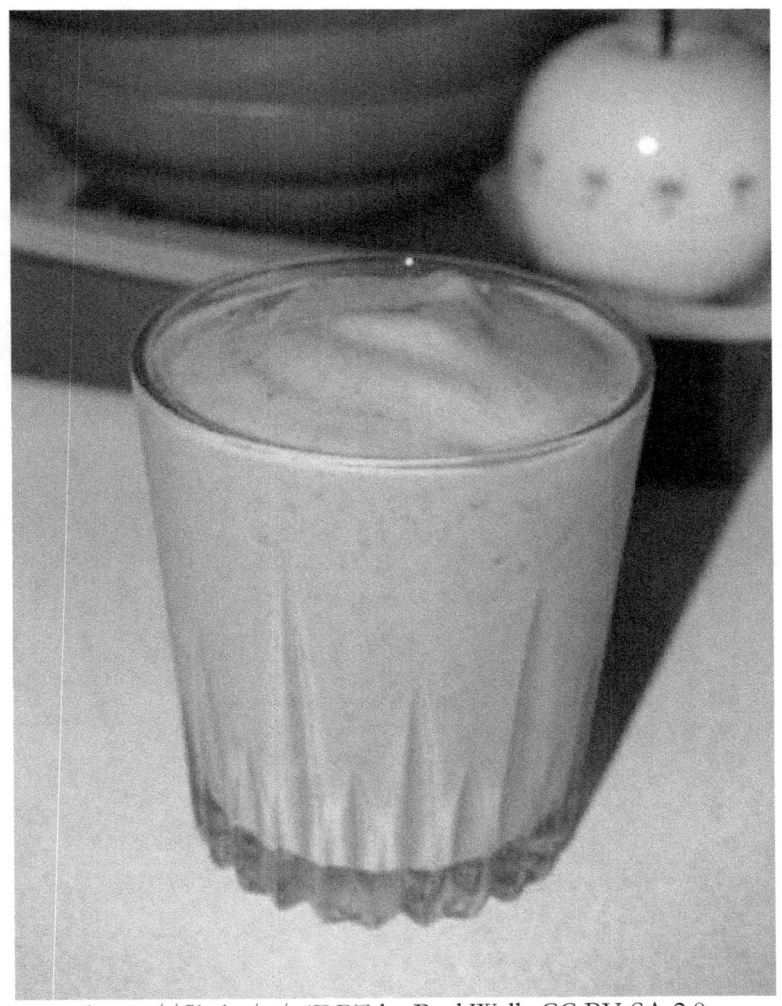

Apple Cashew Cinnamon Smoothie

Serves: 2
Prep Time: 10 minutes

Ingredients:
1 apple, peeled, cored, quartered
2 tbsp cashew butter
½ cup almond milk
½ cup ice

½ tsp cinnamon

Directions:
1. Place ingredients in blender and mix until smooth.

Tomato Kale Smoothie
Serves: 2
Prep Time: 10 minutes

Ingredients:
1 cup low-sodium tomato juice
½ cup kale, washed, chopped
½ cup ice
¼ tsp black pepper

Directions:
1. Place in blender and mix.

Pumpkin Spice Smoothie
Serves: 2
Prep Time: 10 minutes

Ingredients:
1 cup pumpkin, steamed, cooled
½ cup coconut milk
½ cup ice
¼ tsp cinnamon
¼ tsp clove, crushed

Directions:
1. Place in blender and mix until smooth.

MAINS: SOUPS

Creamy Spinach and Bacon Soup
Serves: 4
Prep Time: 10 minutes

Ingredients:
8 cups, washed and chopped spinach
4 slices turkey bacon, cooked and crumbled
1 onion, peeled and chopped
1 cup coconut milk
3 cups low-sodium chicken broth
1 tsp each sea salt and pepper
Olive oil

Directions:
1. Coat 4 qt. slow- cooker with olive oil.
2. Place ingredients in slow cooker and cook on medium for 3 hours.

Creamy Cauliflower Soup
Serves: 4
Prep Time: 10 minutes

Ingredients:
1 cauliflower head
1 can coconut milk
1 cup low-sodium chicken stock
1/4 cup cashews
1 tsp thyme
1 tsp salt
Extra virgin olive oil

Directions:
1. Lightly coat 4 qt. slow cooker with olive oil.
2. Place cashews in blender and crush.
3. Chop cauliflower into florets and place in slow cooker.

4. Add remaining ingredients and mix.
5. Cook on low for eight hours.
6. Using immersion blender, mix until smooth.
7. Sprinkle with your favorite green herb before serving (optional)

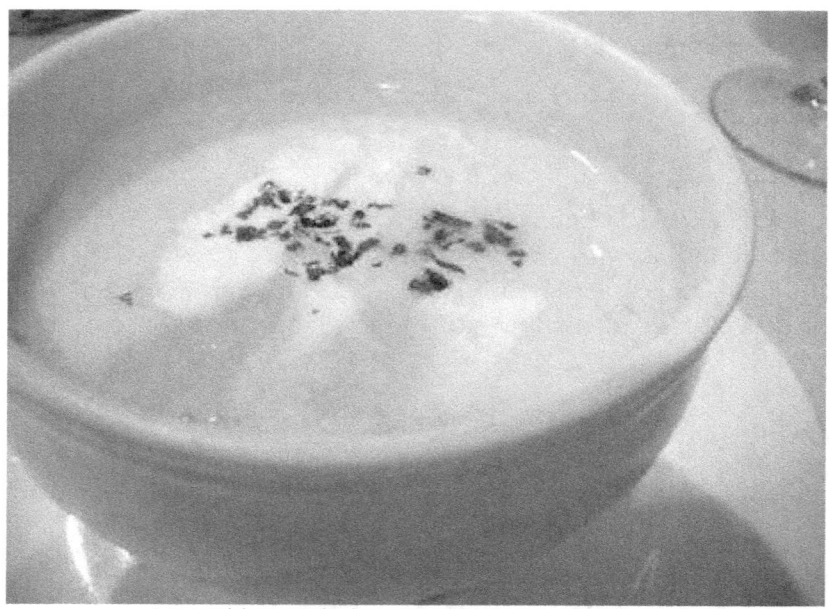

Roasted Red Bell Pepper Harvest Soup

Serves: 6
Prep Time: 10 minutes

Ingredients:
3 red bell peppers, seeded and quartered
2 carrots, peeled and quartered
2 sweet potatoes, peeled and quartered
4 cloves garlic, minced
1 onion, diced
1 cup coconut milk
1 cup water
Extra virgin olive oil

Directions:

1. Preheat broiler and lightly coat roasting tray with olive oil.
2. Place bell pepper, carrot, sweet potato, onion and garlic in roasting tray, drizzle with   oil, and cover with aluminum foil and place in oven for 25 minutes.
3. Heat 2 tbsp olive oil in soup pot, add roasted vegetables, coconut milk, and water   and bring to boil.
4. Reduce heat, simmer for 20 minutes.
5. Using immersion blender, blend until smooth.

Bacon Cauliflower Soup

Serves: 4-6
Prep Time: 10 minutes

Ingredients:

8 cups cauliflower florets
4 strips bacon, cooked and crumbled
1 cup coconut milk 2 cups low- sodium chicken stock
1 tsp salt, pepper
Sprig fresh rosemary
Extra virgin olive oil

Directions:

1. Coat 4 qt. slow-cooker with olive oil.
2. Place ingredients in slow-cooker, cook on medium for 4 hours.
3. Using immersion blender, blend cauliflower soup until nice and creamy.

Turkey Chili

Serves: 4
Prep Time: 10 minutes

Ingredients:

1 lb ground Turkey
1 onion, peeled and diced.
8 cloves garlic, peeled, minced
2 carrots, peeled and chopped
2 celery stalks, peeled, chopped
2 cups tomato purée

2 cups low-sodium chicken stock
1 tsp oregano
1 tsp cumin
1 tsp cayenne pepper
1/2 tsp cinnamon
Extra virgin olive oil

Directions:
1. Heat olive oil in soup pot, sauté garlic, onion and celery.
2. Add ground turkey, brown.
3. Add remaining ingredients, bring to boil.
4. Reduce heat, cover and simmer for an hour.

Creamy Turnip Soup
Serves: 4
Prep Time: 10 minutes

Ingredients:
8 medium turnips, peeled and chopped
1 red chili pepper, chopped
2 green onions, chopped
4 cloves garlic, peeled and minced
3 cups low-sodium chicken broth
2 cups water
1 tsp each salt, black pepper
Extra virgin olive oil

Directions:
1. Heat 3 tbsp olive oil in soup pot; add onion, garlic, chili pepper and sauté for a minute.
2. Add remaining ingredients and bring to boil, reduce heat to medium-low cover, and cook for 30 minutes.
3. Using immersion blender, mix soup until smooth.
4. Sprinkle with your favorite fresh green herbs before serving (optional).

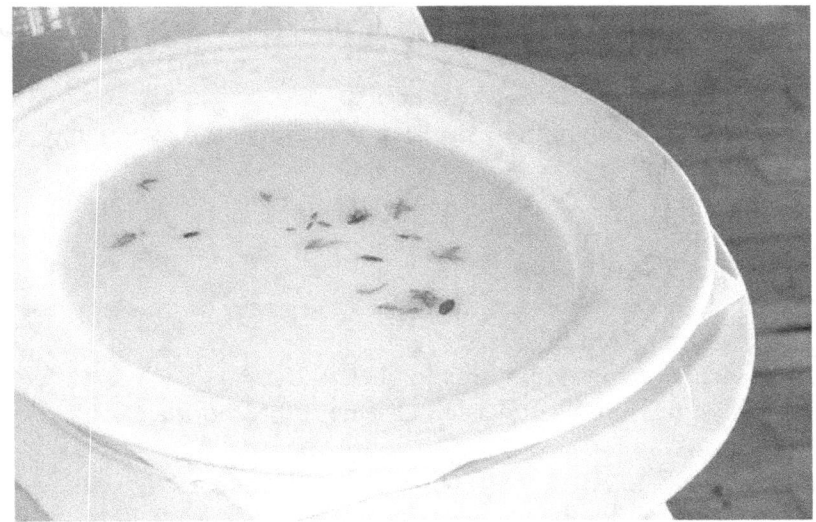

CHICKEN, BEEF, PORK

Rosemary Chicken and Sweet Potato Mash

Serves: 4
Prep Time: 15 minutes

Ingredients:
8 skinless chicken thighs
1 tbsp rosemary
2 lemons, juiced
1 tsp salt, black pepper
Extra virgin olive oil

Sweet Potato Mash
2 sweet potatoes
1/2 cup coconut milk
1 tbsp ghee
1 tsp salt

Directions:
Chicken

1. Mix lemon juice, rosemary, salt and pepper in large glass bowl and place chicken thighs in bowl to marinate overnight if possible or for at least two hours.
2. Preheat oven to 375 degrees, lightly coat roasting tray with olive oil.
3. Place chicken thighs on tray and cook for 30 minutes in oven, turning halfway.
4. Sweet Potato Mash
5. Peel sweet potatoes, quarter and place in steamer for 25 minutes or until tender.
6. Mash sweet potatoes, mix in ghee.
7. Next mix in milk and salt and whip until smooth.

Roast Chicken Breast on Zucchini Toast

Serves: 4
Prep Time: 10 minutes

Ingredients:
4 pieces of 4 oz chicken breasts
4 zucchinis
1 cup fresh basil
1/4 cup cashew
1/4 cup extra virgin olive oil
2 lemons, juiced
1 tsp salt, pepper

Directions:
1. Place basil, cashew, lemon juice salt, pepper in blender and mix into thick marinade.
2. Coat chicken breasts in marinade and allow to sit for an hour.
3. Preheat oven to 375 degrees and coat 2 glass baking trays with olive oil.
4. Place chicken breast in one tray, bake for 20 minutes, baste with marinade at 10 minute mark and turn over.
5. Chop ends off zucchinis and slice in half lengthwise.
6. Place zucchini in second tray and bake for 20 minutes, turning halfway.
7. Place one breast between two zucchini slices and slice on diagonal.

8. You can wrap halves in wax paper to make sandwiches easier to hold.

Blueberry Walnut Chicken
Serves: 4
Prep Time: 10 minutes

Ingredients:
1 lb chicken breast
1 cup blueberries
1/2 cup walnuts
1 cup water
1 tsp each salt and pepper
Extra virgin olive oil

Directions:
1. Cube chicken breasts, place in glass bowl, drizzle with olive oil and sprinkle with salt and pepper.
2. Heat skillet and saute chicken breasts cubes for ten minutes.
3. In frying pan, heat 2 tbsp olive oil, add blueberries, water and bring to boil, add walnuts and continue to cook for five minutes
4. Top chicken with blueberry walnut sauce and serve with green salad of choice.

Curried Chicken on Cauliflower Rice
Serves: 4
Prep Time: 10 minutes

Ingredients:
1 lb chicken thighs
6 cloves garlic, peeled and minced
2 medium onion, peeled and chopped
2 medium tomatoes, chopped
2 cups low-sodium chicken stock
1 cup water
1 tsp cumin
1 tsp curry powder
1 tsp paprika

1 tsp salt, pepper
Extra virgin olive oil

Cauliflower Rice
1 medium cauliflower head
1 cup low-sodium chicken stock
Extra virgin olive oil

Directions:

1. For curry chicken, lightly coat 4 qt. slow cooker with olive oil.
2. Place chicken breast in bottom of slow cooker, add remaining ingredients, and cook on low for 8 hours.
3. Cauliflower Rice
4. Grate cauliflower into rice-like granules.
5. Heat 3 tablespoons olive oil in nonstick pot.
6. Sauté cauliflower for three minutes.
7. Add chicken stock, bring to simmer, cover for five minutes on medium- low.
8. Uncover and sauté for another few minutes until moisture has evaporated.
9. Serve curried chicken on top of cauliflower rice.

Tropical Chicken Skewer

Serves: 2
Prep Time: 10 minutes

Ingredients:

½ lb chicken breast, cubed
½ cup pineapple
1 red bell pepper, seeded
Extra virgin olive oil
1 tsp salt
1 tsp paprika

Directions:

1. Preheat oven to 400 degrees, coat baking tray with olive oil.
2. Place chicken breast in baking tray, drizzle with a little olive oil, and add salt and pepper.
3. Bake for 15 minutes turning half-way.

4. Slice bell pepper into ½" wide strips, slice again horizontally.
5. Alternate chicken breast, pineapple, bell pepper on chicken skewer.

Eggplant Lasagna

Serves: 4-6
Prep Time: 15 minutes

Ingredients:
1 lb lean ground beef
6 cloves garlic, peeled, minced
2 large onions, peeled, diced
3 large eggplants
3 cups tomato purée
1 cup low-sodium beef stock
1 tsp oregano
1/2 tsp paprika
1 tsp salt, pepper
Extra virgin olive oil

Directions:
1. Heat 2 tbsp olive oil in skillet; add garlic onions, sauté for a minute, add ground beef and brown.
2. Add tomato purée, chicken stock and spices, cover and cook on medium-low for 10 minutes.
3. Preheat oven to 400 degrees, lightly coat lasagna tray with olive oil.
4. Chop ends off eggplant and slice vertically into long strips.
5. Place 1/3 of eggplant strips in bottom of lasagna tray.
6. Top with 1/3 sauce mixture, continue layers, cover with aluminum foil and bake in oven for 30 minutes.

Thai Coconut Beef on Squash Noodles

Serves: 4
Prep Time: 20 minutes

Ingredients:
16 oz round steak
1 red bell pepper, sliced

2 cups broccoli florets
1 green onion, chopped
1 cup coconut milk
2 tsp lemon grass
1 tbsp ginger, grated
1 tsp curry powder
1/4 cup coconut oil
1 tsp salt, pepper

Squash Noodles
1 spaghetti squash

Directions:
Squash Noodles
1. Preheat oven to 400 degrees and coat baking tray with coconut oil.
2. Slice spaghetti squash in half, remove seeds, lightly brush flesh with coconut oil, place face down in baking tray and roast in oven for 30 minutes.
3. Remove from oven, using fork remove spaghetti strands from squash halves.

Thai Coconut Curry
1. Heat coconut oil in medium-sized pot; add beef and sauté until browned, remove beef into plate.
2. Add onions, ginger, bell pepper into same pot, sauté for a minute, add broccoli and sauté for another five minutes
3. Add beef back into pot as well as remaining ingredients, save spaghetti squash, reduce heat, cover and simmer for 10 minutes.
4. Serve Thai Beef Curry over spaghetti squash.

Garlic Meatballs with Tomato Basil Salad
Serves: 4-6
Prep Time: 15 minutes

Ingredients:
1 lb lean ground beef
1 medium onion, minced
4 cloves garlic, minced

1 egg
1/4 cup crushed almonds
2 tbsp tomato purée
1 tsp oregano
1 tsp salt, pepper

Tomato Basil Salad
2 tomatoes, sliced
1/4 cup fresh basil, chopped
2 cups green leaf lettuce
2 tbsp extra virgin olive oil
1 lemon juiced
Salt, pepper to taste

Directions:
1. For meatballs preheat oven to 375 degrees and coat baking tray with olive oil.
2. Crack egg into large glass bowl and whisk.
3. Add remaining ingredients, combine well.
4. Using hands roll into 2" balls and place on baking tray.
5. Bake in oven for 20 minutes, turning halfway.

Tomato Basil Salad
1. Mix olive oil, lemon juice, salt, pepper, in large bowl.
2. Toss dressing with tomato, lettuce and serve with meatballs.

Molasses Pork Chops on Cauliflower Purée
Serves: 4
Prep Time: 10 minutes

Ingredients:
4 pork chops, bone-in
6 cloves garlic, peeled and minced
2 medium onion, peeled and chopped
2 cups low-sodium chicken stock
1/4 cup molasses
6 cups cauliflower florets
1 tsp oregano
1 tsp paprika

1 tsp salt, pepper
Extra virgin olive oil

Directions:
1. Lightly coat 4 qt. slow cooker with olive oil.
2. Place cauliflower florets on bottom of slow cooker.
3. Add remaining ingredients, topping with pork chops, then molasses.
4. Cook on low for 8 hours.

Baked Pork Tenderloin with Avocado Chips
Serves: 4
Prep Time: 10 minutes

Ingredients:
1 lb pork tenderloin
2 green apples, peeled, cored and diced
2 avocados, pitted, peeled
1 onion, sliced
1 carrot, peeled and chopped
1 tsp grated ginger.
1 tsp salt, black pepper
1 tsp rosemary
Extra virgin olive oil

Directions:
1. Preheat oven to 375 degrees and lightly coat baking tray with olive oil.
2. Combine salt, pepper, rosemary in tray and roll tenderloin in the dry mix.
3. Place onion, ginger and apples in bottom of baking tray and place pork tenderloin on top.
4. Place in oven for 10 minutes, turn tenderloin over and place back in oven for another 10 minutes.
5. Cover tray with aluminum foil and place in oven for another 20 minutes.
6. While pork is cooking, slice avocado into ½" slices and grill 3 minutes per side, sprinkle with salt.
7. Serve alongside succulent pork.

Italian Sausage and Sweet Peppers

Serves: 4
Prep Time: 10 minutes

Ingredients:
1 lb lean Italian pork sausage
3 red bell peppers, seeded
1 onion, sliced
4 cloves garlic, peeled and chopped
2 tsp oregano
2 tbsp olive oil
Salt and pepper to taste

Directions:
1. Slice sausage into 1/2" discs.
2. Slice bell peppers into strips.
3. Heat 2 tbsp olive oil in skillet, add garlic, onion and stir for two minutes.
4. Add sausage and cook for another 8 minutes, ensuring both sides are browned.
5. Toss in bell peppers and cook for three minutes so that peppers retain some body and replace the feel of a noodle. Season with salt and pepper to taste.

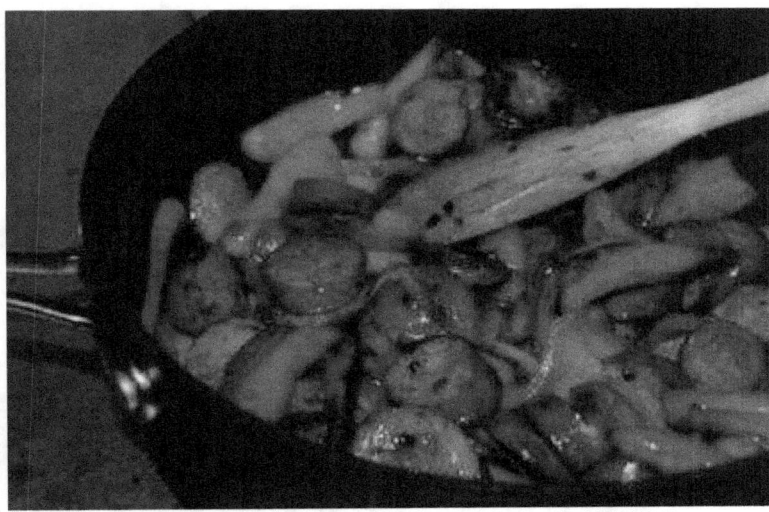

https://flic.kr/p/4tnXCW by Melinda CC BY 2.0

Jalapeno Pork In Peach Cups

Serves: 4
Prep Time: 10 minutes

Ingredients:
2 boneless pork chops
2 jalapeño peppers, seeded, chopped
4 peaches
1 tsp salt, pepper
Extra virgin olive oil

Directions:
1. Preheat oven to 375 degrees and coat baking tray with olive oil.
2. Slice pork into strips.
3. Heat 3 tbsp olive oil in non- stick pan and sauté pork until lightly browned.
1. Add jalapeño, season with salt and pepper sauté for another two minutes, remove   from heat.
4. Slice tops off peaches, remove pit, scoop out a little flesh and place on baking tray
2. Stuff peaches with pork chop mixture, allowing mixture to spill out an inch high over top of peaches.
6. Replace tops on peaches and bake in oven for 10 minutes.

Pulled Pork on Zucchini Toast

Serves: 6
Prep Time: 10 minutes

Ingredients:
2 lbs pork tenderloin
1/2 cup molasses
2 cups puréed tomato
1 cup low-sodium chicken stock
2 tbsp Frank's Red Hot Sauce
Extra virgin olive oil

See Roast Chicken on Zucchini Toast for Zucchini Toast recipe and ingredients.

Directions:
1. Coat slow cooker with olive oil.
2. Place pork tenderloin in bottom of cooker, add remaining ingredients
3. Cook on medium for 4 hours.
4. Shred pork with fork and serve on zucchini toast.

SEAFOOD

Tuna Burgers

Serves: 4
Prep Time: 10 minutes

Ingredients:
450 g (3 cans) Albacore tuna
1 red onion, chopped
1 lemon, juiced
1 egg
3 tbsp almond flour
1/4 cup fresh dill
1 tsp salt, coarse black pepper
Extra virgin olive oil

Eggplant bun
1 eggplant

Directions:
1. Preheat oven to 350 degrees and coat two baking trays with olive oil.
2. Crack egg into large glass mixing bowl and whisk.
3. Add remaining ingredients, save eggplant.
4. Mix together, form into patties and set in baking tray.
5. Place on baking tray and cook for 20 minutes turn tuna burgers halfway.
1. Slice eggplant into 1" slices and place on baking tray, drizzle with olive oil, bake in oven for 20 minutes.
6. Serve tuna burger sandwiched between eggplant slices.

Salmon with Dill
Serves: 4
Prep Time: 10 minutes

Ingredients:
4 x 4 oz salmon fillets
1/4 cup dill
4 tbsp ghee
4 cups arugula
1 onion, sliced
1 lemon, juiced
1/2 tsp salt, black pepper

Directions:
1. Preheat oven to 375 degrees.
2. Heat ghee in large non-stick oven-safe pan, add dill.
3. Place fish in pan, skin- side down and cook for seven minutes.
4. Remove pan from stove and place in oven for another seven minutes.
5. Combine arugula with onion, lemon, salt and black pepper.
6. Serve salmon with salad.

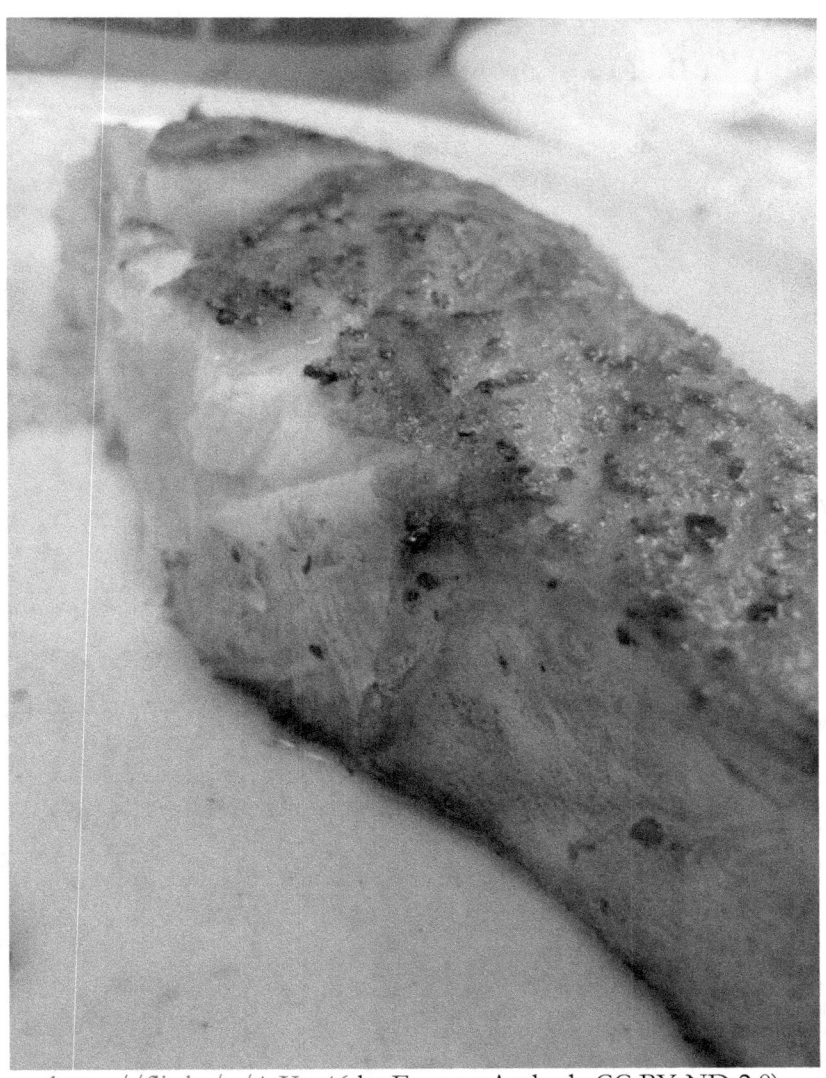

Shrimp in Bell Pepper Pots

Serves: 4
Prep Time: 10 minutes

Ingredients:
1 lb shrimp, peeled, deveined
1 tbsp ghee
4 cloves garlic, peeled, chopped
1 medium onion, peeled, finely diced
4 red bell peppers
1/2 tsp paprika
1 lemon, juiced
1 tsp salt, pepper
Extra virgin olive oil

Directions:
1. Preheat oven to 400 degrees and lightly coat baking tray with olive oil.
2. Slice tops of bell peppers, remove seeds and place on baking tray.
3. Heat ghee in non- stick pan, add garlic, onion, sauté for a minute, add shrimp, sauté   for another minute, add salt, pepper, paprika.
4. Stuff bell peppers with shrimp mixture, drizzle with lemon juice, replace tops and bake in oven for 15 minutes.

Baked Salmon and Arugula Salad

Serves: 4
Prep Time: 10 minutes

Ingredients:
16 oz salmon fillets
2 lemons, sliced into rounds
1 tsp salt, pepper

2 cups arugula
1 cup cherry tomatoes, halved
2 green onions, chopped

3 tbsp extra virgin olive oil
4 tbsp lemon juice
1/2 tsp salt, coarse black pepper

Directions:
1. Preheat oven to 400 degrees, coat baking sheet with olive oil.
2. Place salmon filets on tray skin-side down, sprinkle with salt, pepper, drizzle a little olive oil and place slice of lemon on each fillet.
3. Bake for 15 minutes.

Salad
4. Mix salt, pepper, lemon juice, olive oil in large bowl and toss with arugula, tomato, onion.

Serve salmon alongside Arugula salad

EGGS AND VEGGIES

Spinach Pancakes
Serves: 4
Prep Time: 20 minutes

Ingredients:
Spinach Pancakes
3 cups spinach
1 egg
1 cup almond flour
1/2 tsp salt
Extra virgin olive oil

Directions:
1. For pancakes, combine ingredients with 1 tbsp olive oil.
2. Heat 2 tbsp olive oil in frying pan and pour in approximately 4 tbsp worth of spinach   mixture per pancake.
3. Serve pancake topped with parsley chutney (recipe to follow).

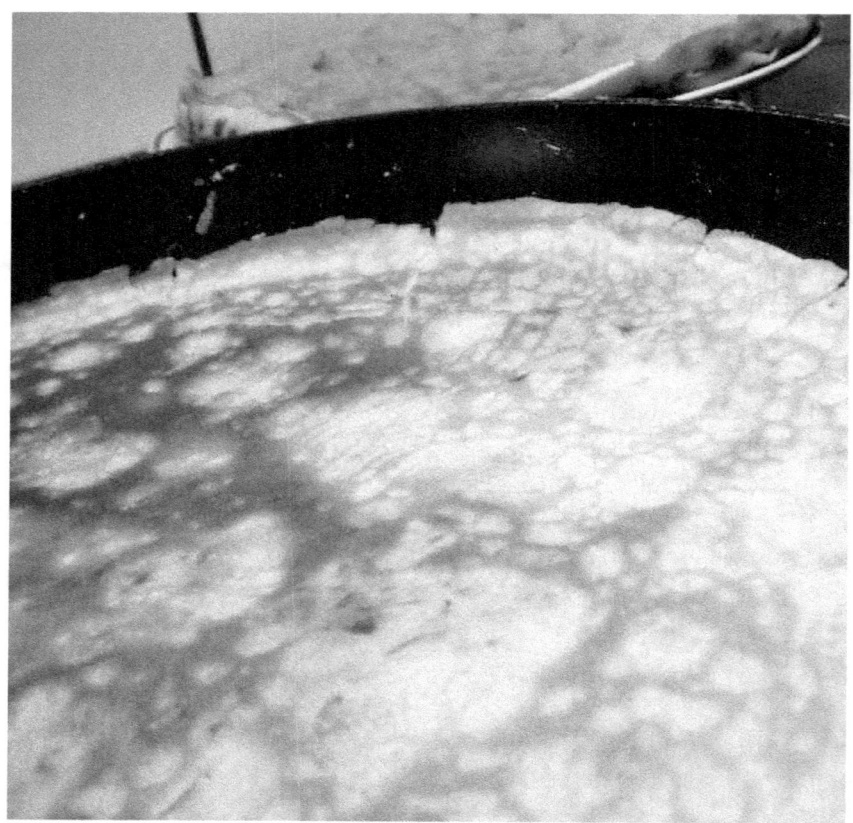

Parsley Chutney
Serves: 4
Prep Time: 10 minutes

Ingredients:
1 green onion, chopped
1 cup parsley, chopped
2 tbsp olive oil
1 lemon, juiced
1 tsp salt, pepper

Directions:
1. For chutney combine ingredients in food processor, pulse for a minute.

Ginger Veggie Spaghetti

Serves: 4
Prep Time: 20 minutes

Ingredients:

1 cup baby carrots
2 cups broccoli florets
1 cup parsnips, chopped
1/2 cup green onion, sliced
1/2 cup low-sodium chicken broth
1 tbsp ginger, crushed
1 tsp each salt, black pepper
1 tbsp coconut aminos
Extra virgin olive oil

Spaghetti
1large spaghetti squash (see Thai Coconut Beef on Spaghetti Noodles for recipe and procedure)

Directions:

1. Heat 2 tbsp olive oil in wok or skillet, add onion and garlic and cook for a minute.
2. Add veggies, ginger and stir- fry for five minutes.
3. Add remaining ingredients and continue to cook for 10 minutes.
4. Remove squash from oven, using fork scoop out spaghetti strings from squash.
5. Toss spaghetti with veggies and serve.

Spaghetti with Creamy Garlic Avocado Sauce

Serves: 4
Prep Time: 10 minutes

Ingredients:

1 avocado, pitted
3 eggs, hard boiled
1 tbsp garlic salt
1 cracked black pepper
1 cup low-sodium chicken stock

Extra virgin olive oil
1spaghetti squash (see Thai Coconut Beef on Spaghetti Noodles for recipe)

Garnish
Handful parsley, chopped

Directions:
1. Place all items in food processor, save squash, blend until smooth.
2. Heat 1 tbsp olive oil in saucepan, pour in blender contents and cook on medium for 10 minutes continually stirring.
3. Toss spaghetti squash with sauce and sprinkle with parsley.

Slow-Cooker Spinach Quiche
Serves: 4
Prep Time: 20 minutes

Ingredients:
8 eggs
4 cups spinach, washed, chopped
1 onion, diced
3 tbsp almond flour
2 tbsp almond milk
Extra virgin olive oil

Directions:
1. Lightly coat 4 qt. slow cooker with olive oil.
2. Mix ingredients and pour into slow-cooker.
3. Cook on low for six hours.

Green Eggs and Bacon
Serves: 2
Prep Time: 10 minutes

Ingredients:
4 eggs

1 cup spinach, chopped
4 slices bacon
1/2 tsp, salt, black pepper
Extra virgin olive oil

Directions:
1. Cook bacon in skillet until browned.
2. Whisk eggs with spinach, salt, pepper.
3. Heat 1 tbsp olive oil in nonstick pan and pour in omelet mixture.
4. Cook for a minute, flip and cook for another few minutes.
5. Enjoy with bacon.

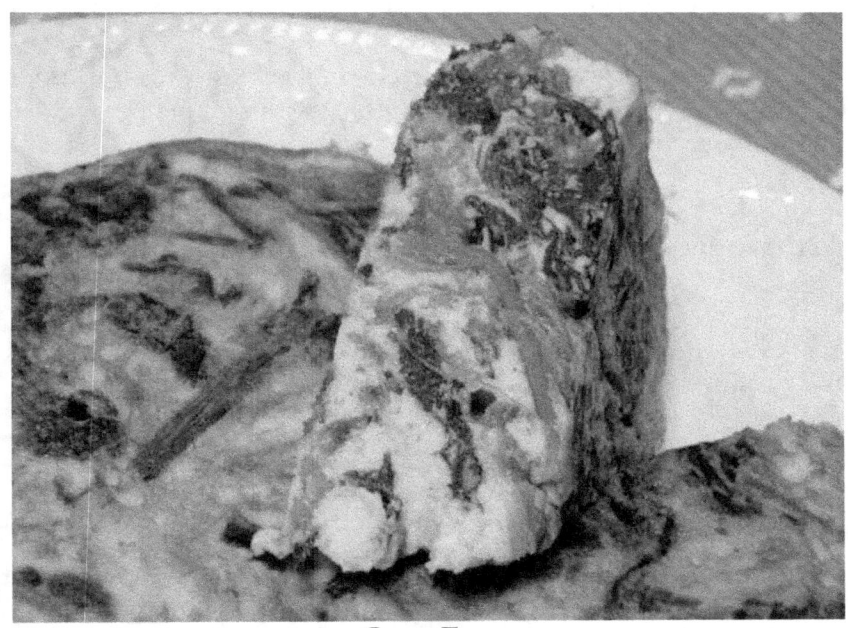

Green Eggs

Egg in Portabella Mushroom bowl

Serves: 4
Prep Time: 10 minutes

Ingredients:

4 Portabella mushrooms, pop off the stem but leave the gills intact
4 eggs
Salt and pepper to taste
Extra virgin olive oil

Directions:

1. Preheat oven to 375 degrees and lightly coat baking tray with olive oil.
2. Place mushrooms on tray, crack one egg into each mushroom, lightly drizzle with olive oil, sprinkle with salt, pepper and bake in oven for 15 minutes.

Rich Avocado-Stuffed Eggs

Serves: 2
Prep Time: 10 minutes

Ingredients:

4 eggs
1/3 avocado, peeled
1/4 tsp paprika
Salt, pepper to taste

Directions:

1. Hard-boiled eggs peel and slice in half.
2. Place egg yolks, avocado, paprika, salt, pepper in food processor and mix until smooth.
3. Spoon egg and avocado back into egg whites.